"Amanda Kingsley is an inte
to earth to liberate people w
forms of shame, aloneness, and limitation. *What I Wish* will be
dog-eared by thousands of badass human beings who feel seen,
free, and alive after having encountered these sacred pages."

> —Kassi Underwood, author of *May Cause Love: An
> Unexpected Journey of Enlightenment After Abortion*
> + host of the Big Energy podcast

"The wisdom in these pages is infinite. It simply is impossible to
quantify the life-changing power of these insights from Amanda
Kingsley. Each message is a force unto itself, but taken all together
they offer a clear way out of the cultural conditioning that traps so
many of us in unjustified stigma. Kingsley writes from personal
experience with the goal of helping others avoid the emotional
struggles rooted in needless shame. Her book is like a map for
finding buried treasure. She shows us all how to discover the
riches of self-assurance that have been with us all along, riches
rooted in our intuitive, responsible, loving decisions about our
reproduction. People who read this book will never have to look
back and wish, but instead will feel free to go forward with the
confidence that is their right."

> —Karen Thurston

"With a frank beauty, Amanda Kingsley's writing offers her
readers both encouragement and direction in claiming the innate
wisdom and power that each of us holds within ourselves. Her
collection of poignant reflections on the experience of abortion is
an invitation to breathe deeply, to feel deeply, and to embrace our
humanity fully."

> —Rev. Katey Zeh, author of *A Complicated Choice:
> Making Space for Grief and Healing in the Pro-Choice Movement*

"Meaning, purpose, gratitude. I devoured this book, not because I have had an abortion, but because I am infertile and never will. Amanda is giving us the book we have waited for since 1973. Her bravery and connection to the authentically real experiences of abortion is necessary if we are to protect the right, improve access, and move beyond the binary of the pro-choice-anti-choice narrative. I am so grateful for her work and her words. Read it and share it with all your friends."

—Dr. Melissa Bird

"At 15-years-old, I had unprotected sex. I didn't get pregnant, but if I did, I would have chosen abortion to avoid the shame evangelical culture put on me.

It's Amanda's book I would have needed because she writes with genuine wisdom, affirming women's worth and denouncing the patriarchal influences of society. Quotable lines throughout the book inspire me to shed shame and break out of Puritan influence. God's unconditional grace flows between Amanda's words, soothing and uplifting.

One for you and one for a friend—*What I Wish* is that kind of book."

—Kara Bohonowicz, KaraBohonowicz.com

WHAT
I WISH

100 love notes to help you survive,
come alive, and thrive after abortion

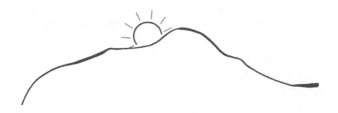

AMANDA STAR KINGSLEY

INTO LIGHT PRESS

Paperback 978-1-957135-00-7
Ebook 978-1-957135-01-4

Into Light Press
www.intolightpress.com

To the babies and the wombs they touched,
your courage does not go unnoticed
or unappreciated.
Your stories are woven into the collective
where they will be cradled
nourished
nurtured
by all of us who have felt the complexity of termination.

Contents

In no particular order, but an order nonetheless:

A note from the author:

I found my way to abortion in my late thirties.
I've known that I wanted to be a mom for as long as I can
remember.

Pregnancy, to me, is still one of the most miraculous and
beautiful human experiences.

Wombs, to me, are magical places filled with power,
purpose, and potential.

I live in a constant state of awe that sperm and egg can come
together and create life inside the human body.
and
I lovingly and gracefully chose abortion.

Abortion was messy.
It was muddled.
It was also a miracle.

My miracle.

Suchlike the miracle of my three living children,
and the pregnancy I carried to miscarriage.

When I chose abortion, I chose me.

I chose my family.
I chose this future.

And I believe
that I also chose her.

Baby Grace.
Our girl here in spirit.
This was how she was meant to be here all along.

She lives in these words—
my work
this life.

And as you read
she also lives in you.

I didn't carry that pregnancy to term,
but I birthed a new me
and together we're thriving.

You are not broken.

People don't break.

Bones break
skin breaks
nails break
and sometimes hearts even feel broken...

But people don't break.

Each of your experiences makes you more whole, not less.
Each of your stories makes you more whole, not less.
Each of your relationships makes you more whole, not less.

Humans are in a constant process of becoming more.

We don't break—
we season
we marinate
we flow
and we RISE.

We do it together.
Together we rise.

You are not alone.

Feeling alone doesn't mean you are alone.

You're telling yourself:
my situation is different
no one is saying what I'm feeling
she is luckier than me
he doesn't understand...

You aren't alone.
You've been taught to believe that
you are alone.

We humans attach ourselves to made-up stories
and most of them are lies.

Believing you're alone gives you permission to stay stuck
permission to be a victim
permission to feel the pain you are feeling.

And it gives someone else your power.

You don't need permission to suffer.
You need permission to heal
to come alive
to thrive.

You need to take back your power.

Abortion is how you protected yourself.

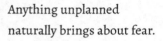

Anything unplanned
naturally brings about fear.

Fear isn't a bad thing;
it is a human thing.

Fear is a survival mechanism.
When we accept that
we can celebrate our fear.
It's on our side.

What we want when we are afraid is to be protected.
Abortion is one of the ways we protect ourselves.

When we don't want what we have
we seek ways to cleanse ourselves of it.

This cleansing doesn't always look and feel good
but we're in it for the long game.

We are in it for the future that we desire.

We protect ourselves by choosing abortion.
This is a mark of our wisdom
not our sin.

Abortion is a choice of instinct.

We choose abortions to be better parents:
to the children we have
to the children we want to have
to this home we call Earth
and this species with which we commune.

Choice is how we care for ourselves.

How we:
nurture our desires
tend to our bodies
and remain faithful to our hearts.

We choose abortion in the interest of the highest good,
and sometimes what's in the interest of the highest good
doesn't feel easy at first.

*Knowing you don't want a baby
is a parental instinct.*

Abortion isn't just about babies.

When we make the decision to abort we're also aborting
the children
the teens
the adults
they would have become.

This doesn't have to be filled with sadness—
it's simply a matter of life.

As mothers we make maternal decisions all the time.

Some fertilize our children into
becoming something,
and some terminate the path they were on.

Every decision matters—
it matters all the way through.

But there is no right or wrong.

Always and only
what's right and wrong for you.

And always happening exactly as it's meant to,
whether we're willing to see that or not.

Call it whatever you want.

Product of pregnancy.
Embryonic tissue.
Fetus.
Baby.

You decide.

You can name her.
You can talk to him.
You can dissociate.

The power is yours.
Your body
your connection
your language.

Words create feelings
feelings create action
action creates results.

Your abortion.
Your life.
Your results.

Hearts don't break.

Hearts ache.
They throb.
They hurt.

But they don't break.

Abortion asked your heart to work extra hard.
The pain you feel is a strengthening
a conditioning
a grooming.

Rest assured your heart has not broken
nor will it break moving forward.

You can let that fear go—
surrender to the sensation
allow it to be nutrient for your growth.

Your heart is malleable,
flexible
adaptable.

It's not broken.

Hearts don't break.
They beat.
And your beat goes on.

Your grief is a result of layered loss.

Grief is a feeling of discomfort accompanying a loss.

After abortions we grieve:
our sense of safety in the world
our trust in—and/or connection to—our bodies
our beliefs about intimacy
our now-changed relationship
the identities we thought defined us.

Grief looks like:
sadness
shock
numbness
denial
powerlessness
fear
anger...

It is as varied as the circumstances that trigger it.

Grief is a normal and necessary part of the
human experience.

It is an invitation to slow down
to explore
to get to know yourself.

When allowed in its fullest expression
your grief will transform into fuel for your future.

It's not just abortion.

You're processing so much more than abortion:

identity
justice
social systems
purpose...

Abortion stirs the pot.

It swirls up all the things in life you thought you could avoid
you thought you didn't have to look at
you thought you could comply with...

The person you used to be
saw the world through different lenses.
Now you have an abortion filter through which to look.

Your eyes are still adjusting.
Your heart is still adjusting.

You are expanding.
The world is a little bigger than you once believed it to be.

Abortion isn't hard.

Hard isn't a fact.
It's a belief system.

We've been programmed to believe
that the choice to abort is hard.
The procedure is hard.
The healing is hard.

But hard is a story.

Choosing to believe something is hard is optional.
It can serve us by validating our feelings.
It can support us in feeling stronger—
if we want it to.

There's nothing wrong with believing something is hard—
if it serves you.

When you're ready
remember that hard isn't a real thing.

Hard is an opinion, just like
right or wrong
good or bad
better or worse.

You decide.

Decision is your power.

Blame won't set you free.

It's natural to want to blame.
But not everything of nature is good for us.

We think blame will make us feel better.
We think it will relieve us
of some of the weight on our shoulders
and in our hearts.

But the only thing it provides
is very temporary relief from your own mind.

Blame shifts your focus,
but it doesn't heal your heart.

Like a knife to the skin, it draws your attention elsewhere—
giving you one more thing to heal.

Your freedom is in acceptance.
Acceptance releases the weight and lightens your load.

It gives you room to take intentional action toward healing
and change.

Decisions can't haunt you.

Decisions are made,
then life moves forward.

The decisions of our past can't haunt us.
The only thing that lives on
are our thoughts about those decisions.

There is an infinite combination of words you can shape into
thought:
Choose intentionally.
Choose purposefully.
Choose lovingly.

Thoughts create feelings.
Feelings create action.
Action creates results.

Results are what you long for.

You long for the life for which you made your choice:
to survive,
to be a better parent,
to get that dream job,
to heal the cracks in your relationship,
to travel, play, nourish, and nurture.

Your freedom isn't locked inside your past decision,
it lives in your present life.

Forgiveness is not a reward.

Most people look for forgiveness
from outside of themselves.
They try to earn it with their actions.

They spend their time and their energy
attempting to prove something
so they can wear forgiveness like a badge.

But forgiveness is a choice.

It's your choice,
and yours alone.

You decide it
you accept it
you believe it
all from within.

The whole world can forgive you,
but until you choose to forgive yourself
you'll always be longing for what you have carried all along.

Be careful with your imagination.

Imagination is a beautiful thing,
but not when you use it against yourself.

Imagination can create or destroy.

Thoughts can bring you to life
or knock the life out of you.

Imagination created everything you see and love—
it also created everything you despise.

In truth
everything is made-up.
Everything was once nothing—
and now it is something.

All of it.

Imagination is at play all around you,
all of the time.

Of course you think about it every day.

In the beginning, abortion can feel ever present—
like a newborn.

Calling to you as you long for sleep.
Waking you with a need for constant attention.
Interrupting your work
your relationships
your social life.

In the ever-swirling thoughts
you hardly recognize yourself or the world anymore.

Nothing has gone wrong.

This is a part of your evolution.
This is a part of your story.

You are becoming the person you were always meant to be.

This isn't the time to push back—
this is the time to surrender.

Get curious.
Listen.
Cherry-pick.
Sculpt.

You are transforming
and you have more power than you've been led to believe.

Life is an ever-changing recipe.
Abortion is an ingredient in the legacy you will leave.

It's not going to go back to "normal."

Normal is a misconception.

We don't get to go back to "normal."
It never really existed.

Normal is this.
Normal is now.
Normal is ever evolving.

Adaption
creation
progression.

LOVE.

The person you were before abortion hasn't disappeared.

She's evolving.

Kiss the hand that holds these words.
Touch the heart that takes them in.
Caress the womb that's taken this journey.

You are the new normal.

There's nowhere to go back to—
forward cradles your opportunity to thrive.

There's nothing to fix.

We live in fix-it times.
Fix-it is a fallout of capitalism.

If there's something to fix
then there's something to sell.

We also live in systematically oppressive times.
Fixing tricks us into believing
we can rise in the hierarchy by being "better."
If one person is "less than"
someone else must be "more."

As women we've been socialized to believe
we aren't good enough.

Our bodies aren't good enough
our ideas aren't good enough
our choices aren't good enough.

Nonsense.
All nonsense.

You weren't broken when you got pregnant,
and you're not broken now.

Liberate yourself by remembering that
you can choose to grow through what you go through—
but doing so doesn't make you any more or less whole.

It makes you more of who you already are.

Regret isn't a bad thing.

Regret isn't inherently bad.
In fact
it can inform future decision-making
in a rich and valuable way.

It's okay to say,
I regret my decision.

It's also okay to regret one abortion and not another.

Regret has no playbook and no rules;
it also has no power.

Shame and guilt don't come from regret;
they come from your thoughts about regret.

Thoughts you can change.

You cannot rewrite your abortion,
but you can rewrite your thoughts.

You decide.

Failure is a sham.

You didn't fail when you were learning to walk.
No one says,
They are learning to walk, but they keep failing.

Your life is a success.

Failure is a made-up story
by people who want to maintain power.

Perspective redefines our lived experiences.

Success is all the parts of you:
all the parts of your story
all the ugly cries and pounding fists
all of it.

Success is love.

And love always says,
Keep going.

Stigma can't hurt you.

Stigma is a set of someone else's thoughts.

Stigma doesn't pay your bills.
Stigma doesn't keep your abusive partner off of you at night.
Stigma doesn't help you raise the kids you already have.
Stigma doesn't launch you into your next promotion.
Stigma doesn't feed the multiplying cells in your womb.

Stigma doesn't get a vote.

It's a set of words and opinions intended to control you,
and you do not need to be controlled.

You know exactly how to run your life.

Stigma shows you the people and places
that want to break you down,
but you are stronger than someone else's beliefs.

YOU are meant for more.
Abortion is a part of your more.

It's okay to be uncomfortable.

Comfort is a beautiful thing:
a resting place
a being place.

But not a growing place.
Comfort doesn't expand you.

Discomfort is where you grow.

Discomfort is a feeling
and it's meant to be a part of your human experience.

We are designed to break open before we bloom.
Abortion cracks us open.

It reveals to us
—and to the world—
a new part of who we are.

It shows us new ways to love
new passages to journey
new places to go.

Discomfort is never the problem.
Our resistance to discomfort
is what sabotages our human experience.

Everything is here to show you something—
discomfort included.

Discomfort is a part of growth.

There's a raw and vulnerable you.

She hides when all is calm—
she rests.

You wouldn't be complete without her.
You need her
but not all the time.

When discomfort slips in,
she awakens.

She nods her head
clears her throat
and gets ready to protect you.

She can't help you when you are in your comfort zone.

It is in your struggle
your pain
your wobble
that she thrives.

Don't push her away.
She is what makes you magic.

Your past is whole and complete.

Nothing you've been through needs fixing.
Telling yourself what is broken
denies its purpose in your life.

Flowers with missing petals aren't broken.
Marriages with arguments aren't broken.
Friendships with disagreements aren't broken.

They are all here to show us a new way to see.

Abortion is part of your whole.
The experience happened for you.

No matter what you do next,
nothing is missing.

It never was,
and it never will be.

Wholeness isn't in what was;
it's in how you see what was.

Trust your feelings.

None of the things you are feeling are bad.
I promise.

They are all here for you.

Relief is here for you.
Shame is here for you.
Grief is here for you.

These feelings are all part of you.
These feelings complete you.

They were a part of you before abortion
and they will be a part of you long after.

The feelings we experience after abortion are complex.
They are supposed to be complex.

They are calling to us
to step deeper into the fullness of who we are.
They are an invitation to become more authentically alive.

Your grief is not forbidden.

Forbidden is an opinion.

Silence after abortion is widespread
but at the mercy of opinion.

Collective opinion doesn't make something more real
it makes it more potent.

You can break the silence.

Grief after abortion is normal.

Grief after all loss is normal:
loss of life
loss of potential
loss of identity...

Our grief feels forbidden
because so many of us suffer quietly,
but hiding doesn't make our pain go away.

It makes it more gnarly.

You have permission to grieve.
It will smooth the edges of your pain.

You don't have to prove anything.

You were born worthy.

Raw, vulnerable, reliant,
and worthy.

In your infancy, you had nothing to prove.
Nor do you now.

Abortion didn't change your value.

It came to remind you that you are human.

Raw, vulnerable, reliant,
and worthy.

You don't have to do anything.
You don't have to be anything.

You are enough.

Exactly as you are.
With a womb full of story
a womb full of strength.

Raw, vulnerable, reliant
strength and worthiness.

You couldn't have been or done any more.

Everything that led you here was enough.
Including you.

You are enough.

You did enough
asked enough
considered enough
tried enough.

I know this to be true because "enough" is a fallacy.

Enough is a lie we're all striving to achieve
but the truth is
there is no enough.
It doesn't exist.

You couldn't have been any more enough then
than you are now.

Enough looks like:
settling in and being
without comparison
without judgment
without disdain.

Only then will you find the freedom you desire for more.

You don't have to _____ .

You don't have to heal.

You don't have to forgive.

You don't have to find purpose in the pain.

You don't have to do anything after your abortion.

But if you want to you can:

learn something new about yourself

learn something new about the world

let go of something you don't want to believe anymore

interrupt an old pattern

build a new life.

There are no explicit rules.

There are no universal expectations.

You get to do you

any way that you want to after abortion.

You don't have to desire peace.

Being at peace with your decision isn't a have-to.
Don't go after anything someone else says you should feel.

You may desire time after abortion to rest
to feel your rage
to contemplate life
to dissect oppression.

This is an important time.
This is part of your growth.

Be with yourself
notice your thoughts
allow your feelings
try on new beliefs.

Discovery is a craving of your humanity.

If along the way you discover peace—
so be it.

It's okay to feel conflicting feelings.

Grief and Relief
Pride and Shame
Trust and Fear

Feeling is freeing.

All the feeling,
the entire human experience.

Conflicting thoughts don't mean we are broken
or that something has gone wrong;
they mean we are human.

Freedom doesn't come from choosing grief or relief;
it comes from allowing both.

Release self-judgment,
release other people's stories,
allow yourself to be fully and complexly human.

It won't be all you think about forever.

There's nothing wrong with you
if all you think about is your abortion.

Some things in life open us up a little wider than others.

If you're still thinking about it
then there's more to explore.

It's whispering
nagging
hollering at you
because it has something to show you.

Believe.
Breathe.
Listen.
Pivot.

Abortion isn't in your thoughts to haunt you—
it's there to enlighten you.

People will see you differently.

That has nothing to do with you,
and everything to do with them.

When you are ready
sharing your story is one of the most powerful ways to heal.

It can set you free
connect you with the collective
ground you in your being.

When you share
people will have opinions.

Some opinions will delight you;
some opinions will shake you.

You get to decide what you make it all mean.

Opinions don't change you.

They help you become who you are meant to be,
who you have been becoming all along.

Don't overthink it.

Let your abortion be what it needs to be.

If it felt transformational
let it transform you.

If it felt unremarkable
let it drift behind you.

If you listen
abortion will tell you
how it wants to integrate into your life.

If you keep listening
it may also evolve over time—
meandering in and out of your consciousness—
exactly how it was meant to all along.

Thinking won't give meaning to your experience.
Only being can do that.

It's okay if it doesn't all make sense yet.

Sometimes it feels like life
gave you a few whirls in a salad spinner.
It's okay to feel dizzy.

For most people
abortion isn't one of those take-your-time decisions.

Things can happen fast—
it can feel upside down
sideways
and leave you wondering who you even are.

Take a breath.
Feel your feet on the ground.

You're still you—
same hands
same toes
same heart.

Still you—
only now, you have a beautiful opportunity
to get to know even more of yourself.

Your thoughts will change over time.

Time doesn't heal all wounds.

Emotional pain after abortion is sourced in our thoughts.
What we think is what we feel.

In time, thoughts change.
Changing thoughts, changing feelings.

Tend to the gift that is your mind.
Your mind is where you will find peace;
your mind is where you will find freedom.

Your mind is both the simplest
and the most complex tool you have.
Use it wisely, or it will use you.

Feed it nourishing content
surround it with loving company
be patient with it
but forever diligent.

You were programed to survive,
but you were born to thrive.

It's not black-or-white.

The world has taught us that things are supposed to be
black-or-white
right or wrong
good or bad.

What we actually feel in most of our lives is much less clear.

We're not confused—
we're human.

It's not messy—
It's complex.

Abortion isn't right or wrong.
It simply is.

Abortion isn't good or bad.
It simply is.

We don't have to painfully straddle the ravines of:
relief and regret
shame and confidence
denial and resistance
peace and distress.

We can walk, curiously, back and forth between the two.

We can allow all of it.
Every intricate detail.
One perfectly imperfect moment at a time.

This is a season.

This time
this space
this experience—
it is a part of the living whole.

Someday you will look back
and reflect on the season of your abortion.

Your perspective will have changed.
Your beliefs will have changed.
Your feelings will have changed.

This truth is inevitable.
Being human will always include change.

It's tempting to resist that which we do not like,
but allowing it all is where you will find peace.

This season serves a purpose.
Watch curiously as it evolves.
Be with yourself as you evolve.

No one needs to hear your story
more than you.

How we tell our story matters.
How we hear our story matters.

Nothing is fixed—
especially not your abortion story.

Story elicits feeling
and feeling is fuel.

You pick:

I couldn't have his baby.
or
I chose to release my tie to him.

I had no choice.
or
I chose for a reason.

My birth control failed.
or
I didn't get the results I expected.

Our stories are where we cultivate light
or darkness.

Abortion isn't fixed—
our thoughts about it determine
whether we live in the dark
or we live in the light.

If you listen, you will be guided.

You don't have to understand in order to receive.
We are always being spoken to.

Those thoughts that swoop in
and puzzle you with perfection
perhaps they are from sources you cannot see or touch.

Maybe that coincidence
isn't a coincidence at all.

Your future self
a passed loved one
your soul baby
God...
You are guided.

You are not alone.

Ask.
Listen.
Act.

You have nothing to lose
and everything to gain.

Let go and surrender.

There will be times when you want to rewind—
give it all back
skip the lesson
pretend it never happened.

Let go.
Surrender.
Be here now.

Resistance has you fighting reality.
Surrender will lead you to growth.

Your life has a flow.
It's moving with the entire universe in perfect alignment.
Resistance thwarts the flow.
Surrender sanctions it.

Letting go can feel scary,
acceptance can be mistaken for giving up,
but you were born for this.

Release your grip.
Surrender to the reality that is your abortion.

In this alignment you will shine.

*Life is happening **for** you.*

Abortion didn't happen to you.
It happened for you.

No,
you contend.

Yes,
I hold.

Abortion is your coat of many colors.
It is your humanity.
An expression of your wombhood.

Abortion has invited you to feel all the feelings.
The feelings are for you.
All of them.

They make you stronger.
They make you wiser.
They make you fuller.

They are here for you.
Life is happening *for* you.
Abortion included.

Don't leave yourself behind.

Don't leave behind the piece of you
who believed abortion was the right choice.
Let her be your guide.

She had a wish.
She had a dream.
She had desires that haven't disappeared.

Life stirred up around her,
but she's still there.
She wants you to find her and remember her.

Work with her
not against her.

You are a team.

Your life crew includes all the versions of yourself
all the decisions that have been made
all the lessons that have been learned
all of you.

You can slow down now.

It felt rushed.
Who's to say rushed was a bad thing.
Rushed may have been
exactly how you needed to make that decision.

You can slow down now.
You can catch your breath.
You can make a plan.

Abortion happened
AND
you're still here
here with a future
here to live the life you chose.

Some things in life move fast
and others slow;
you don't always get to decide.

But you can always choose.
Choose to feel.
Choose to heal.

Choose this very moment you are in and ask,
Now what?
How do I want to show up now?

Love yourself anyway.

There will be people who don't like your choice—
you can love yourself anyway.

There will be people you judge you—
you can love yourself anyway.

There will be people who take your choice personally—
you can love yourself anyway.

People will be people;
you only get this one lifetime to love yourself:

Fully.
Completely.
Unconditionally.
Even imperfectly.

You don't have to like all of you.

You don't like all the parts of your mother.
You don't like all the parts of your partner.
You don't like all parts of your best friend.

It's okay to love someone and not like everything about them.

Give yourself grace.

The whisper inside of you
that wishes you were a little different
it's showing you where to hold space for your growth.

Love emerges where you nurture it.

Seek out the places in yourself where love already resides.
Lean in where your love lands softly and with compassion.

Be in those places for as long as you need to.
Help them grow.

They are where you'll find your freedom and naturally
expand who you are meant to be.

You can trust yourself.

Stop looking to your past for evidence that you can be
trusted with important things.
Your past only exists in your present thoughts.

Life wasn't given to you to get *right*.
There exists no right.
Only right now.

Right is inside you.

It can't be determined by someone else's beliefs
someone else's judgments
or someone else's playbook.

Right isn't proven by what you did—
it is determined by what you do next.

Life was given to you to play
to explore
to feel
to get messy.

Trust is built within.

Trust yourself
to keep showing up
to keep believing
to purposefully and compassionately keep going.

Reunite with your body.

You lost touch when your mom told you
you shouldn't eat that third cookie
at age ten.

You lost touch when your
friends in middle school had
less belly in their bikinis.

You lost touch when you told him
NO
and he fondled you anyway.

You lost touch when all those
fertility treatments failed.

Or maybe
you didn't lose touch until you were blindsided
by the unplanned pregnancy.

Now is the time to let all of that go.

Not to forget it
but to redefine it.

Now is the time to reunite.

Love her.
Caress her.
Whisper sweet nothings
into every nook and cranny of her miraculous shape.

She needs you now more than ever.

She needs you to rekindle the flame you had
before the world started telling you lies.

Take the shoulds out of your womb.

You were socialized to believe that it's your duty,
—and should be your desire—
to raise children.

It's a lie that holds up the patriarchy.
Inside this lie, women have been
providing unpaid labor for hundreds of years.

Free your womb from other people's agendas
by following your heart.

Your body is not an incubator,
and your arms are not obligated to society.

Abortion is a loss.

A passed pregnancy,
a passed opportunity,
a past identity...

But it's also a gain.

A gained freedom
a gained direction
an exercised independence.

Shoulds indicate an oppression with which
your heart will never align.
They don't belong in your womb or in your life.

You're gonna be okay.

It might not feel like it,
but you're gonna be okay.

I know that because you are human
and if you made it this far
you are a warrior.

You have beaten the odds.
Your life is a treasure.

Abortion wasn't a sentence,
it was an invitation.

Okay doesn't always look pretty.
It's not a statue.
It's a state of being.
And it's ever evolving.

All of the ups
downs
and sideways are you being okay.

Freedom comes in embrace.

Get out there.
Go be okay.

Go with all of you
all of the ups
downs
and sideways.

I'm here too.
Here being okay with you.

Your body remembers.

Historically, carrying pregnancies to term
and raising healthy children
came with a boatload of challenges.

Those times have passed.

Most of us have clean water.
Most of us have enough food.
Most of us understand germ theory.
Most of us have access to medical care.

BUT

There's DNA in you that remembers harder times.
There once was a time when the womb carried
the survival of the human species.

There's an ancient whisper in you that says,
Pregnancy and childbirth are a treasured miracle.

You can hear that whisper from the past
and choose abortion for your present.
The survival of the species is no longer your burden to bear.

You are not your ancestors
and what you do with your womb
does not define your worth.

Your body is perfect.

All that body shaming
the way society told you
that you weren't good enough as you are
the way they sold someone else's image
as more desirable than yours
it's here in abortion too.

For centuries you've been sold the lie that
someone else's body is better than yours
even their womb.

The stigma that's surrounded abortion
keeps us in shackles of shame.

And because we're not talking about abortion as a humanity
we don't know that other wombs look just like ours.
Other wombs have stories too.

Your body is perfect.
Neither your pregnancy, nor your abortion
changed that.

*Your decision does not
create your reality.*

Decisions do not determine your well-being.

The way you feel
the things you think
the results unfolding all around you—
they have nothing to do with your decision
and everything to do with your mind.

You chose abortion because you wanted to feel something:
Freedom—from an abusive partner.
Relief—from the discomfort.
Possibility—for your future.

Those feelings don't just happen from a procedure.
The decision to abort
does not create freedom, relief, or possibility.

All of those things are created in your mind.
You have to cultivate them.

There has never been a better time than now
to decide how to feel on purpose.

What you want matters.

It mattered when you chose abortion
and it matters now.
What you want will always matter.

Even when you don't listen to it—
it matters.

There have been
and will be
times when what you want
gets swept away in other people's dreams
other people's fears
other people's beliefs,
but that does not mean anything about you.

Be in a relationship with your own desire:
get to know her
play with her
dance with her
honor her.

Communicate with your wants
as you would a child in your care.

Listen.
Negotiate.
Collaborate.
And eventually see that she is her own energy.

You've been called here—
not to manipulate and manage your desire
but to allow it
nurture it
and hold space for it to come to life.

Don't underestimate the power of knowing what you don't want.

It's okay if you're still not sure what it is that you do want.
Knowing what you don't want is invaluable.

There exists no one without the other.

You made a decision knowing that you didn't want to carry
that pregnancy to term.

Your brain may try to trick you into thinking
you made a mistake—
that's only because it doesn't know how to grieve.

Your brain is confused.
Grief is a feeling, and your brain thinks in thoughts.
It's looking for a plan.

Abortion is a loss:
a lost pregnancy
a lost identity
a lost dream...

Let your heart do the work.
Connect with your highest self.

You knew what you didn't want;
now trust that what you do want will reveal itself to you.

Make room for your life to unfold
by identifying all the things you do and do not want.

There's nothing missing.

Empty is an illusion.

Your baby is not missing.
Not gone.
They haven't left you.

The manifestation of that pregnancy
was not a breathing human being,
but don't be mistaken—the space has been filled.

Creation occurred.

A new you
a new perspective
a new belief...

Pregnancies don't just birth babies—
they create life.

This life you have in front of you
is the fruit of that conception.

Honor it.
Nourish it.
Nurture it.

Nothing is missing.
Quite the opposite.

*It's okay to feel like you are,
or were, not yourself.*

The you before choosing abortion
didn't know that this you existed.

She didn't know because abortion
wasn't something for which she planned.

There was no time to prepare
get acquainted with
or adapt to a new identity.

But there is time now.

You weren't supposed to feel like yourself.
How could you?

Past you hadn't been introduced to future you.
Make room for that now
and everything changes.

Listen, feel, accept
and everything changes for the better.

This is how we evolve.
This is how we thrive.

Your feelings aren't isolated to abortion.

Abortion didn't give you shame.
It didn't serve you a plate of grief.
It didn't riddle you with regret.

All those feelings are a part of you.
They always have been.
They always will be.

Abortion gave you an opportunity to explore them
accept them
allow them.

Abortion has invited you to step into your fullest
most beautiful human self.

In acceptance
the world is at your fingertips.

Feel shame and
you realize it has no power over you.

Experience grief and
you understand it is a flavor of your love.

Witness your regret and
you free yourself from your fears.

Abortion doesn't produce your feelings
it reminds you that you have them.

All your feelings are fertilizer.

Feeling is never a mistake.

You were divinely created to feel.
All of it—
even when it doesn't make sense.

Relief & Grief.
Shame & Pride.
All of it—
even when it feels conflicting.

Never a mistake.

Feelings are an invitation to explore.
They are the nutrient for your growth.

Like compost
sometimes they reek
they burn
they decompose and give life.

Thriving
nourishing
vibrant
LIFE.

What you plant in the soil of your life
will grow with your feelings.

Be tender and intentional with your gardening.

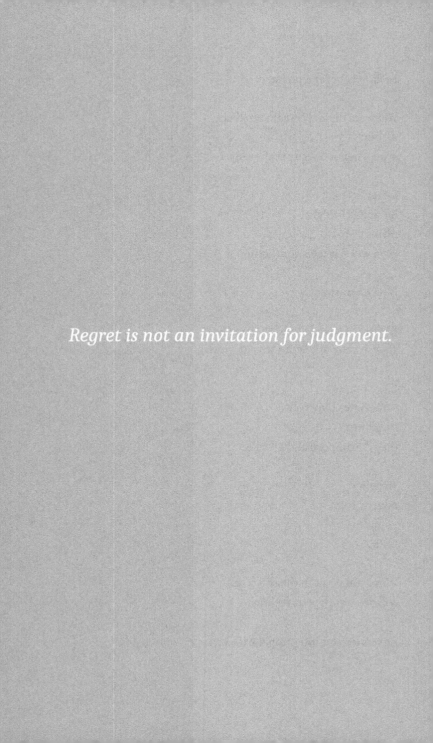

Regret is not an invitation for judgment.

You can regret your decision
and love yourself *and* your life.
You cannot regret your decision
and hate yourself *and* your life.

Regret is not a measure by which to judge.

Strength and courage are available to you.
Right now.
Always.

The choice to regret is in your control.
You have the power.
You've had it all along.

Freedom looks like having your own back.
Freedom looks like bravely stepping forward.

Freedom looks like courageously being with what is
and deciding what to make it mean.

Regret offers an invitation to redefine yourself.

Abortion didn't empty you.

Finding joy in your life after abortion
doesn't replace the child you could have had.
Joy honors the experience you did have.

Your joy shines light on the ways you've grown
the struggles you overcame
the evolution you were meant to experience all along.

We don't choose to thrive after abortion in order
to fill a space left by an unborn soul.
We choose to thrive for ourselves—
sometimes in honor of that unborn soul.

There's no actual emptiness after abortion.
There's no hole in your heart.

I know it can feel that way
but abortion didn't empty you—
it filled you.

Filled you with opportunity
filled you with wisdom
filled you with light.

Your cup is actually overflowing.
You just have to be willing to shift your perspective
and see it that way.

You are not a sinner;
you are a savior.

Sinners have one thing in mind,
themselves.

To sin is an act of the ego;
It is to put your needs at the peak of an imaginary hierarchy,
and to believe that all we have is this very moment of time.

Saviors are visionary.
Saviors think beyond constructed blinders.
They believe in something bigger
something brighter
something far greater than a moment in time.

You are a savior.

You chose:
YOU, future, family, the unknown.

What you chose was so much bigger than your ego.
Keep choosing.

Just because it's harder to see
does not mean your vision has disappeared.

Just because other people can't see it
does not mean it's not there.

You are not selfish.

Abortion was for you
and:
abortion is for families
abortion is for communities
abortion is for souls who weren't ready to come all the way in.

Choosing abortion takes courage.

Sometimes, what's in the highest good
doesn't feel good up front.

Abortion is an expression of strength
wisdom
compassion
generosity
presence...

You are allowed to own all of that.

Living into the fullest expression of you
is the least selfish thing you can do for the planet.

You can't be forgiven
for a mistake you didn't make.

There are moments when it all feels like a nightmare.

Desperate for relief
you beg for forgiveness—
anything that might make the pain stop.

Solace is destined to come
but it will arrive with acceptance
not forgiveness.

Abortion was always meant to be a part of your story.
There is no need for forgiveness in a perfectly executed plan.

Abortion wasn't a mistake; it was a summon
calling you into your life
calling you into your purpose
calling you into your fullness.

Forgiveness is an illusion.

Your life is here
now
this way
as it's always meant to be.

Balance doesn't always feel balanced.

Balance comes in seasons.

Winter is going to feel imbalanced if you wake up
expecting to experience summer at the very same time.

It's easy to be turned away by the word balance
when you are expecting everything all at once.

Life is more like a series of
ins and outs
ups and downs.

Allow your grief to be grief as long
as it needs to remain that way.
Trust that the natural way of things
will bring a shift in experience.

It's okay to feel unbalanced.
It's perfectly human.

Scan out.
Feel into the whole.
Life might actually be more balanced than you think it is.

You don't owe anyone anything.

Abortion isn't a debt you have to pay back.
It's not a life sentence you are doomed to carry.
And it's definitely not a mark on your sleeve.

You don't owe anyone
an explanation
a justification
or an apology.

Abortion is yours
to do with as you please.

Other people's expectations reflect their beliefs.
They get to decide what to do with their abortions
not yours.

Your body
your choice
your freedom.

Possibility is not responsibility.

At the moment of conception, your world changed.
Your womb became a chamber of new possibility.

But we don't have to say yes to every possibility
that presents itself to us.

We have agency.
We have choice.
We are in control.

In the moment of termination, your world changed again.
Your life became a chamber of new possibility.

Same agency.
Same choice.
Same control.

You get to decide what to say yes to.

Always—
new possibilities
are always accessible.

You get to decide what it means.

After abortion, our thoughts can
swirl
cycle
and torment us.

Birth control can't be trusted.
People can't be trusted.
I can't be trusted.

Brains are always looking for a way to categorize and catalog
our experience,
but as clever as they are
they don't always have our best interest in mind.

We get to decide;
we can put our brains to work for us
not against us.

We get to believe anything we want to believe.

We get to decide.

Abortion showed us what to trust
who to trust
and how to trust.

Your past has gifted you your future.

Some gifts don't come in pretty blue boxes with bows.

Some gifts come with bleeding wombs
and follow-up appointments.
They look like scars to the untrained eye.

Should you choose to see it
abortion showed you your beliefs
your dreams
your feelings
your love.

There was always more to see;
abortion invited you to look closer.

The book you wanted to write, it will be fuller now.
The lips you dream to kiss, they will taste sweeter now.
The legacy you want to leave, it will reach more people now.

But all of this
only when you choose to widen your perspective
and start unwrapping the gifts that you once saw as scars.

Beliefs are products of our imagination.

Every thought you've ever heard about abortion
was constructed in the mind of a human being.

Some thoughts you've kept.
They turned into beliefs.

Some thoughts you've let go.
You gave them no sticking power.

All this
consciously or unconsciously
by choice
by will.

Beliefs are words strung together
in a way that makes sense to the human brain.

One not more important or impactful than another—
until the human brain decides for it to be so.

When we understand that beliefs are simply a product of
our imagination
we realize that we have the power to change them.

With this power
anything is possible.

Don't give away your power.

Choose your thoughts wisely.
That's where your power lies.

Shit happens:
good shit,
bad shit.

If you are human, shit happens.

Power is in your mind.
Your mind controls your future.
The future.

No matter the circumstances—
you can rise.

In sadness, you can choose to elevate.
In celebration, you can choose to elevate.

You are human,
and humans are here to *grow*.

Abortion is asking us to choose growth.
The world is asking us to choose growth.

Growth is power.

Choice is your superpower.

Choosing abortion was not a mistake.
It was a sacred use of your power.

Evolution asks us to keep choosing:

Choose to take care of your body.
Choose to take care of your heart.
Choose to take care of your mind.

Choose who to tell
who to trust
who to heal with...

Our lives keep going
and our choice continues to be our superpower.

Yield your choice like a glowing sword.
Swing intentionally.
Know when to rest.
Claim victory beyond your suffering.

You don't have to let it go.

Letting it go is for arguments and old socks.

You don't have to let your abortion go.

If you want, you can carry it with you
like a freckle
or a stretch mark
a gold locket
or a special key.

It's yours to do with as you please.

It is a part of you
and no one else gets to decide how you do you.

The womb is designed to release what no longer serves it.
It does this most months of our lives.

But it was also designed to hold our deepest,
most intimate treasures.
It carries the seeds for our fertile blooming.

Abortion is a part of our bloom.

Remembering is how we grow.

Forgive and forget is dreadful life advice
for people who want to grow.
Remembering is how we develop ourselves.

Honor your abortion.

Remember who you are.
Reintegrate yourself with your new perspective.
Reinvent yourself.

Live the life you made your choice for,
and if you can't remember what it was,
make something up.

You are in control.
Your life is lived one choice after another.

We choose, we feel, we adapt, and we grow.
This is how we thrive.

There's plenty of time.

No one wins a race for healing the fastest
sharing the most
creating the biggest splash
after abortion.

There are also no prizes for longest-kept secret
or most dues paid.

Unlike babies
abortion stories gestate at all different lengths.

The birth of a new you
won't come with contractions
cervical dilation
and pushing.

It will come with
feeling
adapting
and growing into the fullest
most whole version of yourself.

There's plenty of time,
and like a pregnancy, only you get to decide what to do with it.

*Your thoughts about your abortion
are not isolated.*

We are inherently whole beings.
Abortion included.

Nothing we believe or experience
can be fully extracted
from the complexity of our existence.
Abortion also included.

Unresolved feelings:
grief
shame
guilt
regret—
they seep into all parts of our lives.

When we suffer in one place, we suffer in all places.
When we heal in one place, we heal in all places.

Abortion gifts us opportunity to embrace the fullness of our
human experience and heal with holistic intention.

When we accept all the feelings of our experience
and step intentionally into our growth,
we give ourselves permission to live more vibrant lives.

Lives that exist with a knowing
that we can feel anything and thrive forward.

You've been invited to become something.

Abortion, should you choose to accept it
is an invitation to become something new.

There are a handful of bridges
we may cross as human beings.
Bridges that, in crossing
transform us.

Falling in love.
The loss of a dear friend.
Chronic illness or physical impediments.
Becoming a parent.
Abortion.

Bridges aren't good or bad, per se.
They simply are.
They are a path between two places.

Transformation happens when we emerge from something
by choice or by default
as an entirely different version of being.

Many of us ignore the invitation to evolve.

We are so anxious to get past our pain and return to normal
that we relinquish the greatest opportunity of our lives.

We miss the opportunity to serve the highest calling
of our humanity—the invitation to grow.

Now you know.

You didn't know it would feel like this.
Now you know.

We're not supposed to know all the things ahead of time.
We're supposed to know them when we know them.

So now you know.
Who are you now that you know?

The kind of person who:
writes books
moves to new countries
changes careers
feels all the feels...

You won't know until you know—
and the only way to find out is to try.

Try.
Learn.
Grow.

This is the human experience.

Be careful with what you believe.

You came into this world raw and ready to learn;
your brain
a fertile ground for planting.

You learned love
but you also learned hate.
You learned pleasure
but you also learned pain.

You marinated in all the beliefs of your family
your friends
your culture.

Shaped by your surroundings,
you formed beliefs about:
body image
worth
purpose.

Some messages
you didn't even know were taking root in your mind
but root they did.

Now that you're an adult
it is your job to weed.

You get to decide what beliefs serve the future you desire.

Abortion consumed you,
and it completed you.

Sure, it took some time.
Sure, it took some brainpower.
Sure, it took your attention from other things.

It consumed you.
And it completed you.

This is the you
that you were always meant to be.

Right here.
Right now.

You didn't realize it before,
but you are living, breathing proof of it now.

When your life comes to a close
you can look back
you can see purpose in each of your journeys.

But you don't have to wait—
you can start seeing that purpose now.

Shame keeps us small.

Abortion is a part of your evolution.

Life is full of decisions:
we decide
we learn
we evolve.

There is no wrong way to evolve.
There is no wrong way to grow.

Abortion gave you information.
What you do with that information is in your control.

It showed you who you are
what you're capable of
what you desire
how to live into a future of which you'll be proud.

Shame robs you of your future,
and your freedom is in your honor.

Honor your abortion.

Honor your feelings.
Honor your decision.
Honor your desire.
Honor your future.

Honor you.

Abortion is an act of radical liberation.

We feel shame when we perceive ourselves
to be isolated or left out.

We're biologically programmed to want to fit in;
it's a part of our survival strategy.

To our primal brain, fitting in equals
food,
shelter,
and love.

But the human species is long past its struggle for survival.

The bulk of our shame in the 21st century is learned.

You don't have to be religious
to have been programmed for shame.
Religious and oppressive hierarchy
is what most of our modern culture was built on.

Long before you were born
women's sexuality was labeled dangerous
and subjected to mass oppression and control.

When we choose to abort
we reclaim our bodies and liberate our sexuality.
The shame you feel is a cracking open
of hundreds of years of bad programming.

Release your shame, and you break the bonds of oppression.

Your future is your do-over.

What's done is done.

Your abortion only exists now in yo⌐
reinforced by your spoken word.

Memories are not sculpted in stone—
they are malleable.

With words, you can change your entire experience:

It was a struggle.
It was an opening.

I wish it were different.
I am making the future different.

I don't know who I am.
I am learning who I am.

You don't get an abortion do-over,
but your future doesn't care.

Future you
desires growth
she thrives in expansion
and you are only one thought away
from making her dreams come true.

*You've been given the tools
to face new challenges.*

I can do hard things.
I can have my own back.
I can slow down.
I can love myself in all the ways I've been craving from others.

Savor these lessons.

These are the tools that will land you the promotion
help you find your life partner
guide you to create new things.

What you've been looking for your whole life
is already within—
you were born with the ultimate all-in-one software.

Your mind is the most valuable thing you own,
and no one can take that from you.

You are here.
You are reading.
You are whole.

The world is at your fingertips.

Your brain wants something to do.

Abortion comes layered.

Your brain is trained to excavate the layers
and detect meaning.

Brains like meaning.

Oddly,brains don't care
what meaning we assign to our experiences—
they just want to make sure there is one.

They want to know where to catalog every piece of our lives.
Life events without meaning
feel naked and exposed to the untrained mind.

You can choose.
You can create meaning.
You can decide what to make it all mean.

Your intention will sculpt your future.

Abortion made me stronger.
Abortion made me wiser.
Abortion was the new beginning I had been searching for.

You can choose—and change your mind.
Brains are malleable.
Beliefs are not permanent.

Think for your highest good.

Choose badass, not broken.

Your life will never return to what it was.
It's okay to feel overwhelmed or confused by that.
You don't have to know what's coming next.

If you look close enough
you'll notice that part of you feels a little broken
but part of you feels a little badass.

In every moment, you can choose broken
or you can choose badass.

Start thinking outside the box.

If you can move through an abortion—
what else is possible?
Who else might you be?
What more might you be able to endure
in honor of love and purpose?

Abortion made you wiser.
Abortion made you braver.
Abortion brought you here
where you get to keep choosing badass.

Your joy will be greater.

No one can know the capacity
to which they can experience joy
until they know the capacity
to which they can experience pain.

Abortion is a door—
an invitation to feel more joy.

Life offers us many doors to walk through—
each an opportunity for expansion.

To open ourselves to a richer life
we have to open ourselves to all of it.

The darkness
and the light.

Where there is one,
the other will follow.

*Trying not to think about it
does not make it go away.*

Our life experiences are the skeleton of our future.

We can't wish away what once was.

Whether or not we like it
each of our life events is a part of our foundation.

We can turn our heads and look the other way
but our past always follows.

With love
attention
and acceptance
we can turn each piece of our past
into a pillar of our future:
a lesson learned
a truth revealed
an opportunity delivered.

What we try to hide from
always has a way of finding us.

What we greet courageously and heal through
becomes a light we shine on the rest of the world.

Your soul will never lose its shimmer.

Some days the world feels a little grayer than others.

Today may be one of those days
but remember
your soul is filled with ever-present light.

It is part of an extended web.

It arrived in this body on a mission
and nothing can take away its glow.

Every day we can choose to survive
or we can choose to thrive.

Your soul *always* wants to thrive.

You are directly connected to
the struggling mother in Tanzania
and the celebrity artist in Hollywood.

There is oneness between us.
A tie that binds us.
An energetic connection that weaves through all life.

Your soul is as bright and sparkly
As the most glittering light.

You cannot do anything to change that.
Your opportunity lies in how much of it
you choose to share with the world.

Abortion is how you parented that child.

All of our children are here to teach us something.
Our relationship is mutual.

Some might tell you that your baby had no voice
but they are mistaken.

Souls who choose wombs marked
Pregnancy NOT Desired
know exactly what they are here for.

Anyone who tells you otherwise
does not give enough credit
to the spiritual or human experience.

Not all pregnancies are meant to deliver breathing babies.

Some are testing grounds for souls dipping their feet
in the human form.
Some are meant to deliver fuller
more expanded women.

All pregnancies are opportunities for growth.

To be a parent is to choose love
even when it feels like the hardest thing in the world.

Abortion is an expression of love.

You're not that special.

It's true.
And it's great news.

I know you feel alone.
I know you feel unique.
I know you feel different.

But you're not that special.
Not in that way.

The complexity of your feelings
the loneliness
the confusion—
it's all normal, typical
and expected.

What will make you special is how you rise.

Your strength
your story
your ability to turn darkness into light—
that's what makes you special.

Abortion isn't special
but living purposefully and intentionally after abortion
is more than special.

It's exceptional.

You can choose to be exceptional.

The desire to please isn't wrong.

It's natural for it to hurt
when you think you can't give someone
what you think they want.

A baby
a partner
a friend
a community.

Human beings are givers.
The desire to please isn't wrong.

And
we offer the greatest change in the world when we
give first to ourselves, then to others.

Our impact is far greater from a full cup than from
an insatiable, ill-conceived desire to make everyone happy.

The power hidden in a termination
invites us to live from our own full cup and have faith
that it's the most powerful thing we can do for humanity.

*It wasn't theirs to decide,
and it isn't theirs to heal.*

Unplanned pregnancy happened to you
and for you.
Abortion happened to you
and for you.

You wanted someone else to make the choice,
but it wasn't theirs to make.

You want someone else to "fix it",
but it's not theirs to fix.

These feelings are yours to feel.
This life is yours to live.

You get to learn.
You get to grow.

Your body,
your choice,
your future.

Take back your power with your willingness to be in this
moment
exactly as it is,
exactly as you are.

You can love people
who don't know how to support you.

Our hearts open when we recognize that sometimes
we expect people to give to us
in ways we don't yet know how to give to ourselves.

It's okay that they don't know how to support you.
Like you, they are learning.

You have an opportunity to model compassion
in the very way you desire it most right now.

Love yourself:
your imperfections
your weaknesses
your confusion
your inadequacy
your pain...

Love it all.

It is what makes you whole.

You can reject the people
who don't know how to support you
or you can accept the calling to model self-reliance
in a way that the world has never seen
and is craving to learn.

*Trust people
to be able to handle your truth.*

The way people react to your truth
is not a reflection on you—
it's a reflection on them.

Give them a chance to grow
a chance to expand
a chance to hold space for your story.

Make room for people to surprise you.

Trust yourself to stay steady
come back to your center
stand strong in your path.

Do not let the world tell you who you are supposed to be.
Show them who you are
and invite them to exist beside you.

In the end, there is no one truth
only yours
theirs
and mine
woven together on this human journey called life.

Keep looking—and start creating.

You're not crazy.
The choices *have* been slim.

There's a gaping hole in after-abortion care
and the reason you haven't found what you're looking for
might be that you're the one who's meant to create it.

Your story, your experience
your voice is what the world needs.

It's okay if you wobble;
the ground is rocky.

It's okay if you slip;
the slopes are slick.

Don't turn back.
Keep going.

Heal yourself.
Then get down and dirty
and create something that will leave a legacy.

Create something that will help someone—
something you wish you had when you were in the dark.

Loving yourself isn't a requirement.

There's no rule that says you have to love yourself.

Love is complex.
It's raw and nuanced
and quite frankly it's unstable.

Instead of choosing to love yourself always
you can choose to have your own back.

Commit to falling back in love
even after you fall out.

Relationships are fickle things.
Especially fragile is the one we have with ourselves.

Commit to remember that
perfection isn't the destination.

It's okay to wonder who you are—how you got here
or if you even like yourself anymore.

Wondering is part of the pleasure.
Wondering itself is freedom.

Commit to the wonder.
Be determined to stay by your side—always.

On a path led by curiosity—the chances of falling in
love with yourself again and again are really quite high.

Keep asking.

When you find yourself wondering—
What was the point of my abortion?
What was the purpose?

Know that you asking the question itself
IS the point.

The meaning of life isn't in the answers we find;
it's in the questions we ask.

You don't have to know why today,
and you might not know why tomorrow.
Keep asking.

The asking unrolls a red carpet of discovery.
It's where you will discover who you are
and where you'll create who you want to be.

Be the one.

When what you want doesn't exist
create it.

When what you wish for feels impossible
go for it anyway.

When the world is on fire all around you,
find relief in the depths of your soul.

What if your abortion happened
so that you can be an example of what's possible?

We don't break down barriers with what already exists.
We break them down with what hasn't yet been created.

You can be the creator.
Your abortion can be the catalyst.

You are the meaning.

You want it to mean something.
You want to know it was all for a purpose.

Humans like to understand things.
We like to deconstruct
and to put back together.

We think that if we search long enough
and in the right places, it will all make sense.

In some ways that's true,
but what makes sense was there all along.

We are the meaning;
our evolution is the purpose.

We can't see that until the fear dissipates.

When we release our judgments
feel our feelings
and decide on purpose
we see that abortion happened for us.

It came to show us more of who we really are.
It came to remind us that we are complex creatures
on a journey to love and be loved in all the ways.

What we greet courageously and heal through becomes a light we shine on the rest of the world.

Acknowledgments

To all of us.

To all of you who send me your stories, grace me with your gratitude, and challenge me to think outside the box and outside the outdated narratives. Every time you listen, read, and connect with me, you fuel a change in the world we've waited far too long to see. You are a part of the evolution of reproductive justice.

To my family: my husband, my children, my parents— all who held me up with their love and support through both my abortion and the birth of my life's work, including this book. In so many indescribable ways, you are my light.

To my Papa who always left one thing amiss as a way of saying "I was here."

To the practitioners who made my abortion not only possible, but comfortable. Your commitment to our wellbeing feels like love.

To the women who helped me make this book come alive on paper. Kara Bohonowicz, Emily Stone, and Leah Kent, this book would not be here without your love and support.

And especially to Baby Grace, February 2017–March 2017, my tiny abortion miracle. I knew as soon as you came, there was a reason. I see now that the immaculate IUD removal was your work of art—your pathway to leave a legacy. The world will be forever touched by your complexly beautiful being.

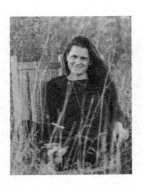

About the Author

Amanda Kingsley is Certified Feminist Life Coach and the host of the *Speaking Light Into Abortion* podcast. She helps people who've had abortions step into the lives they made their choices for.

Her signature program, *Birthing a New You*, guides participants through the post-abortion identity shift. It's where she helps her clients feel to heal, accept and adapt, and when ready, grow into their thriving futures.

She's been featured in *Mothering* magazine, on the *UnF*ck Your Brain* podcast, and on the stage of The Life Coach School. Before her own abortion at age 38, she spent years in the reproductive health field supporting all outcomes of pregnancy and reproductive health.

Connect with Amanda on Instagram @amandastarkingsley or at her website **www.amandastarkingsley.com**

Refuse to be used as a weapon.

Complex feelings after abortion have nothing to do with whether or not safe abortion should be accessible to everyone.

The fact that we experience sadness does not mean we shouldn't have had abortions.

The fact that we wonder what babies would have felt like in our arms does not mean we shouldn't have had abortions.

The fact that we experience shame for having needed an abortion does not mean we shouldn't have abortions.

Abortion doesn't exist in a bubble of standard feelings.
It comes with the full range of emotions and is different for everyone.

Let's refuse to be used as weapons against abortion access.
Let's define our discomfort as a tribute to the strength we now carry now because we had abortions.